AF255454

The Complete Diabetic Meal Prep Cooking Guide

Fast and Irresistible Recipes To Boost Your Metabolism And Burn Fat

James Dale

implied. Readers acknowledge that the author is not engaging in the rendering of legal, financial, medical or professional advice. The content within this book has been derived from various sources. Please consult a licensed professional before attempting any techniques outlined in this book.

By reading this document, the reader agrees that under no circumstances is the author responsible for any losses, direct or indirect, which are incurred as a result of the use of information contained within this document, including, but not limited to, — errors, omissions, or inaccuracies.

Table of contents

Carnitas

Servings: 2

Cooking Time: 50 Minutes

Ingredients:

- Bay leaves (1)
- Garlic (1 clove slivered)
- Oregano (.25 tsp)
- Garlic powder (.25 tsp)
- Adobo seasoning (.25 tsp.)
- Low-sodium vegetable broth (.25 c)
- Cumin (.5 tsp.)
- Roast (1 lb.)
- Chipotle pepper with adobo sauce (1)

Directions:

1. Set your Instant Pot cooker to sauté.
2. Season the pork as desired before adding it to the Instant Pot cooker and cooking each side for about 5 minutes. Remove the pork from the pot and set aside to cool.
3. With the help of a sharp knife, make a 1-in. incision in the pork that is deep enough to accept the garlic slivers.
4. Add additional seasonings to the pork as desired, rub the mixture into the meat.

5.   Add the broth, bay leaf and the chipotle pepper to the Instant Pot before placing it in the Instant Pot cooker pot and sealing the lid of the cooker. Choose the high-pressure option and set the time for 50 minutes.

6.   Once the timer goes off, select the instant pressure release option and remove the lid. Remove the pork and shred using a pair of forks.

7.   Return the pork to the Instant Pot cooker and allow it to soak up any remaining juices, taking care to remove bay before doing so.

Nutrition Info: Protein: 20 grams Carbs: 12.2 grams Fiber: 11.9 grams Sugar: 11.2 grams Fats: 7.5 grams Calories: 320

Air Fryer Roast Beef

Servings: 3

Cooking Time: 45 Minutes

Ingredients:

- 3-1/2 lbs. beef roast
- 2 tbsps. olive oil
- 1 tbsp. rosemary
- 1/2 tbsp. garlic powder
- 1/2 tsp fresh ground rugged black pepper

Directions:

1. Adjust the temperature of the air fryer to 360°F
2. Mix herbs and oil on a plate. Roll the roast in the blend on the plate to ensure that the entire surface of the beef is covered.
3. Set the beef in the air fryer basket. Establish the timer for 45 mins for tool-rare beef, 51 mins for the tool. Examine the beef with a meat thermostat to see if it is done to your liking.
4. Cook for extra 6-minute periods if you like it cooked a lot more. Keep in mind that the roast will undoubtedly remain to prepare while it is relaxing.
5. Eliminate the roast from the air fryer and put on a plate, cover with lightweight aluminum foil. Allow it to rest for 10 minutes before serving.

Nutrition Info: Calories: 666 kcal; Carbs: 0.3g; Fat: 54g; Proteins: 43g

Pork Chops With Grape Sauce

Servings: 4

Cooking Time: 25 Minutes

Ingredients:

- Cooking spray
- 4 pork chops
- ¼ cup onion, sliced
- 1 clove garlic, minced
- ½ cup low-sodium chicken broth
- ¾ cup apple juice
- 1 tablespoon cornstarch
- 1 tablespoon balsamic vinegar
- 1 teaspoon honey
- 1 cup seedless red grapes, sliced in half

Directions:

1. Spray oil on your pan.
2. Put it over medium heat.
3. Add the pork chops to the pan.
4. Cook for 5 minutes per side.
5. Remove and set aside.
6. Add onion and garlic.
7. Cook for 2 minutes.
8. Pour in the broth and apple juice.
9. Bring to a boil.

10.   Reduce heat to simmer.

11.   Put the pork chops back to the skillet.

12.   Simmer for 4 minutes.

13.   In a bowl, mix the cornstarch, vinegar and honey.

14.   Add to the pan.

15.   Cook until the sauce has thickened.

16.   Add the grapes.

17.   Pour sauce over the pork chops before serving.

Nutrition Info: Calories 188 Total Fat 4 g Saturated Fat 1 g Cholesterol 47 mg Sodium 117 mg Total Carbohydrate 18 g Dietary Fiber 1 g Total Sugars 13 g Protein 19 g Potassium 759 mg

Pork Roast

Servings: 2

Cooking Time: 3 Hours

Ingredients:

- Coconut oil (1 T)
- Water (2 c)
- Portobello mushrooms (5 sliced thin)
- Garlic (2 cloves smashed)
- Onion (.5 chopped)
- Celery (1 rib)
- Pepper (.5 tsp.)
- Pork roast (1 lb.)

Directions:

1. Start by adding the garlic onion and celery to the Instant Pot cooker pot before adding in the water and then the roast, before seasoning as desired.
2. Place the Instant Pot cooker pot into the Instant Pot cooker and seal the lid. Choose the high-pressure option and set the time for 60 minutes.
3. Once the timer goes off, choose the instant pressure release option
4. Set the roast aside and place the vegetables and resulting broth into a blender and blend well.

5. Place the roast back in the Instant Pot cooker, seal the cooker and allow it to cook for 2 hours under high pressure, this will help to render the fat and ensure the edges are crisp.

6. When the timer goes off, use the instant pressure release option and transfer the roast to a serving dish.

7. Turn the Instant Pot cooker to the sauté setting before adding in the coconut oil. Once it is heated, add in the mushrooms and allow them to cook for 5 minutes. Add in the gravy from the blender and let it reduce until desired thickness is achieved.

8. Top roast with gravy prior to serving.

Nutrition Info: Protein: 23.8 grams Carbs: 13.2 grams Fiber: 9 grams Sugar: 2.2 grams Fats: 3.5 grams Calories: 360

Stuffed Chicken Breasts Greek-style

Servings: 4

Cooking Time: 20 Minutes

Ingredients:

- 4 oz. chicken breasts, skinless and boneless
- ¼ cup onion, minced
- 4 artichoke hearts, minced
- 1 teaspoon oregano, crushed
- 4 lemon slices
- What you will need from the store cupboard:
- 1 cup canned chicken broth, fat-free
- 1-1/2 lemon juice
- 1 tablespoon olive oil
- 2 teaspoons of cornstarch
- Ground pepper
- Salt, optional

Directions:

1. Take out all the fat from the chicken. Wash and pat dry.
2. Season your chicken with pepper and salt.
3. Pound the chicken to make it flat and thin.

4.   Bring together the oregano, onion, and artichoke hearts.

5.   Now spoon equal amounts of the mix at the center of your chicken.

6.   Roll up the log and secure using a skewer or toothpick.

7.   Heat oil in your skillet over medium temperature.

8.   Add the chicken. Brown all sides evenly.

9.   Pour the lemon juice and broth.

10.   Add lemon slices on top of the chicken. Simmer covered for 10 minutes.

11.   Transfer to a platter. Remove the skewers or toothpick.

12.   Mix cornstarch with a fork.

13.   Transfer to skillet and stir over high temperature.

14.   Put lemon sauce on the chicken.

Nutrition Info: Calories 224, Carbohydrates 8g, Fiber 1g, Cholesterol 82mg, Total Fat 5g, Protein 21g, Sodium 339mg

Shredded Beef

Servings: 2

Cooking Time: 35 Minutes

Ingredients:

- 1.5lb lean steak
- 1 cup low sodium gravy
- 2tbsp mixed spices

Directions:

1. Mix all the ingredients in your Instant Pot.
2. Cook on Stew for 35 minutes.
3. Release the pressure naturally.
4. Shred the beef.

Nutrition Info: Calories: 200 Carbs: 2 Sugar: 0 Fat: 5 Protein: 48 GL: 1

Classic Mini Meatloaf

Servings: 6

Cooking Time: 25 Minutes

Ingredients:

- 1 pound 80/20 ground beef
- ¼ medium yellow onion, peeled and diced
- ½ medium green bell pepper, seeded and diced
- 1 large egg
- 3 tablespoons blanched finely ground almond flour
- 1 tablespoon Worcestershire sauce
- ½ teaspoon garlic powder
- 1 teaspoon dried parsley
- 2 tablespoons tomato paste
- ¼ cup water
- 1 tablespoon powdered erythritol

Directions:

1. In a large bowl, combine ground beef, onion, pepper, egg, and almond flour. Pour in the Worcestershire sauce and add the garlic powder and parsley to the bowl. Mix until fully combined.
2. Divide the mixture into two and place into two (4") loaf baking pans.

3.   In a small bowl, mix the tomato paste, water, and erythritol. Spoon half the mixture over each loaf.

4.   Working in batches if necessary, place loaf pans into the air fryer basket.

5.   Adjust the temperature to 350°F and set the timer for 25 minutes or until internal temperature is 180°F.

6.   Serve warm.

Nutrition Info: Calories: 170 Protein: 14.9 G Fiber: 0.9 G Net Carbohydrates: 2.6 G Sugar Alcohol: 1.5 G Fat: 9.4 G Sodium: 85 Mg Carbohydrates: 5.0 G Sugar: 1.5 G

Skirt Steak With Asian Peanut Sauce

Servings: 4

Cooking Time: 15 Minutes

Ingredients:

- ⅓ cup light coconut milk
- 1 teaspoon curry powder
- 1 teaspoon coriander powder
- 1 teaspoon reduced-sodium soy sauce
- 1¼ pound skirt steak
- Cooking spray
- ½ cup Asian Peanut Sauce

Directions:

1. In a large bowl, whisk together the coconut milk, curry powder, coriander powder, and soy sauce. Add the steak and turn to coat. Cover the bowl and refrigerate for at least 30 minutes and no longer than 24 hours.

2. Preheat the barbecue or coat a grill pan with cooking spray and place the steak over medium-high heat. Grill the meat until it reaches an internal temperature of 145ºF, about 3 minutes per side. Remove the steak from the grill and let it

rest for 5 minutes. Slice the steak into 5-ounce pieces and serve each with 2 tablespoons of the Asian Peanut Sauce.

3. REFRIGERATE: Store the cooled steak in a reseal able container for up to 1 week. Reheat each piece in the microwave for 1 minute.

Nutrition Info: Calories: 361 Fat: 22g Saturated Fat: 7g Protein: 36g Total Carbs: 8g Fiber: 2g Sodium: 349mg

Roasted Pork Loin With Grainy Mustard Sauce

Servings: 8

Cooking Time: 70 Minutes

Ingredients:

- 1 (2-pound) boneless pork loin roast
- Sea salt
- Freshly ground black pepper
- 3 tablespoons olive oil
- 1½ cups heavy (whipping) cream
- 3 tablespoons grainy mustard, such as Pommery

Directions:

1. Preheat the oven to 375°F.
2. Season the pork roast all over with sea salt and pepper.
3. Place a large skillet over medium-high heat and add the olive oil.
4. Brown the roast on all sides in the skillet, about 6 minutes in total, and place the roast in a baking dish.

5.   Roast until a meat thermometer inserted in the thickest part of the roast reads 155°F, about 1 hour.
6.   When there is approximately 15 minutes of roasting time left, place a small saucepan over medium heat and add the heavy cream and mustard.
7.   Stir the sauce until it simmers, then reduce the heat to low. Simmer the sauce until it is very rich and thick, about 5 minutes. Remove the pan from the heat and set aside.
8.   Let the pork rest for 10 minutes before slicing and serve with the sauce.

Nutrition Info: Calories 368 Fat: 29g Protein: 25g Carbs: 2g Fiber: 0g Net Carbs: 2g Fat 70%/Protein 25%/Carbs 5%

Meatballs In Tomato Gravy

Servings: 6

Cooking Time: 30 Minutes

Ingredients:

- For Meatballs:
- 1 pound lean ground lamb
- 1 tablespoon homemade tomato paste
- ¼ cup fresh cilantro leaves, chopped
- 1 small onion, chopped finely
- 2 garlic cloves, minced
- ½ teaspoon ground cumin
- 1/8 teaspoon salt
- Ground black pepper, as required
- For Tomato Gravy:
- 3 tablespoons olive oil, divided
- 2 medium onions, chopped finely
- 2 garlic cloves, minced
- ½ tablespoon fresh ginger, minced
- 1 teaspoon dried thyme, crushed
- 1 teaspoon dried oregano, crushed
- 3 large tomatoes, chopped finely
- Ground black pepper, as required
- 1½ cups warm low-sodium chicken broth

Directions:

1. For meatballs: in a large bowl, add all the ingredients and mix until well combined.
2. Make small equal-sized balls from mixture and set aside.
3. For gravy: in a large pan, heat 1 tablespoon of oil over medium heat.
4. Add the meatballs and cook for about 4-5 minutes or until lightly browned from all sides.
5. With a slotted spoon, transfer the meatballs onto a plate.
6. In the same pan, heat the remaining oil over medium heat and sauté the onion for about 8-10 minutes.
7. Add the garlic, ginger and herbs and sauté for about 1 minute.
8. Add the tomatoes and cook for about 3-4 minutes, crushing with the back of spoon.
9. Add the warm broth and bring to a boil.
10. Carefully, place the meatballs and cook for 5 minutes, without stirring.
11. Now, reduce the heat to low and cook partially covered for about 15-20 minutes, stirring gently 2-3 times.
12. Serve hot.
13. Meal Prep Tip: Transfer the meatballs mixture into a large bowl and set aside to cool. Divide the

mixture into 6 containers evenly. Cover the containers and refrigerate for 1-2 days. Reheat in the microwave before serving.

Nutrition Info: Calories 248 Total Fat 12.9 g Saturated Fat 3 g Cholesterol 68 mg Total Carbs 10 g Sugar 4.8 g Fiber 2.5 g Sodium 138 mg Potassium 591 mg Protein 23.4 g

Garlic-braised Short Rib

Servings: 4

Cooking Time: 2 Hours, 20 Minutes

Ingredients:

- 4 (4-ounce) beef short ribs
- Sea salt
- Freshly ground black pepper
- 1 tablespoon olive oil
- 2 teaspoons minced garlic
- ½ cup dry red wine
- 3 cups Rich Beef Stock (here)

Directions:

1. Preheat the oven to 325°F.
2. Season the beef ribs on all sides with salt and pepper.
3. Place a deep ovenproof skillet over medium-high heat and add the olive oil.
4. Sear the ribs on all sides until browned, about 6 minutes in total. Transfer the ribs to a plate.
5. Add the garlic to the skillet and sauté until translucent, about 3 minutes.
6. Whisk in the red wine to deglaze the pan. Be sure to scrape all the browned bits from the meat from

the bottom of the pan. Simmer the wine until it is slightly reduced, about 2 minutes.

7.   Add the beef stock, ribs, and any accumulated juices on the plate back to the skillet and bring the liquid to a boil.

8.   Cover the skillet and place it in the oven to braise the ribs until the meat is fall-off-the-bone tender, about 2 hours.

9.   Serve the ribs with a spoonful of the cooking liquid drizzled over each serving.

Nutrition Info: Calories: 481 Fat: 38g Protein: 29g Carbs: 5g Fiber: 3g Net Carbs: 2g Fat 70%/Protein 25%/Carbs 5%

Chicken & Spinach

Servings: 4

Cooking Time: 13 Minutes

Ingredients:

- 2 tablespoons olive oil
- 1 lb. chicken breast fillet, sliced into small pieces
- Salt and pepper to taste
- 4 cloves garlic, minced
- 1 tablespoon lemon juice
- ½ cup dry white wine
- 1 teaspoon lemon zest
- 10 cups fresh spinach, chopped
- 4 tablespoons Parmesan cheese, grated

Directions:

1. Pour oil in a pan over medium heat.
2. Season chicken with salt and pepper.
3. Cook in the pan for 7 minutes until golden on both sides.
4. Add the garlic and cook for 1 minute.
5. Stir in the lemon juice and wine.
6. Sprinkle lemon zest on top.
7. Simmer for 5 minutes.
8. Add the spinach and cook until wilted.

9.   Serve with Parmesan cheese.

Nutrition Info: Calories 334 Total Fat 12 g Saturated Fat 3 g Cholesterol 67 mg Sodium 499 mg Total Carbohydrate 25 g Dietary Fiber 2 g Total Sugars 1 g Protein 29 g Potassium 685 mg

Air Fried Chicken With Honey And Lemon

Servings: 4

Cooking Time: 50 Minutes

Ingredients:

- The Stuffing:
- 1 whole chicken, 3 lb
- 2 red and peeled onions
- 2 tbsp olive oil
- 2 apricots
- 1 zucchini
- 1 apple
- 2 cloves finely chopped garlic
- Fresh chopped thyme
- Salt and pepper
- The Marinade:
- 5 oz honey
- juice from 1 lemon
- 2 tbsp olive oil
- Salt and pepper

Directions:

1. For the stuffing, chop all ingredients into tiny
   pieces. Transfer to a large bowl and add the olive

oil. Season with salt and black pepper. Fill the cavity of the chicken with the stuffing, without packing it tightly.

2.   Place the chicken in the Air Fryer and cook for 35 minutes at 340 F. Warm the honey and the lemon juice in a large pan; season with salt and pepper. Reduce the temperature of the Air Fryer to 320 F.

3.   Brush the chicken with some of the honey-lemon marinade and return it to the fryer. Cook for another 70 minutes; brush the chicken every 20-25 minutes with the marinade. Garnish with parsley, and serve with potatoes.

Nutrition Info: Calories: 342; Carbs: 68g; Fat: 28g; Protein: 33g

Honey Mustard Chicken

Servings: 4

Cooking Time: 12 Minutes

Ingredients:

- 2 tablespoons honey mustard
- 2 teaspoons olive oil
- Salt to taste
- 1 lb. chicken tenders
- 1 lb. baby carrots, steamed
- Chopped parsley

Directions:

1. Preheat your oven to 450 degrees F.
2. Mix honey mustard, olive oil and salt.
3. Coat the chicken tenders with the mixture.
4. Place the chicken on a single layer on the baking pan.
5. Bake for 10 to 12 minutes.
6. Serve with steamed carrots and garnish with parsley.

Nutrition Info: Calories 366 Total Fat 8 g Saturated Fat 2 g Cholesterol 63 mg Sodium 543 mg Total Carbohydrate 46 g Dietary Fiber 8 g Total Sugars 13 g Protein 33 g Potassium 377 mg

Greek Chicken Lettuce Wraps

Servings: 4

Cooking Time: 8 Minutes

Ingredients:

- 2 tablespoons freshly squeezed lemon juice
- 1 teaspoon lemon zest
- 5 teaspoons olive oil, divided
- 3 teaspoons garlic, minced and divided
- 1 teaspoon dried oregano
- ¼ teaspoon red pepper, crushed
- 1 lb. chicken tenders
- 1 cucumber, sliced in half and grated
- Salt and pepper to taste
- ¾ cup non-fat Greek yogurt
- 2 teaspoons fresh mint, chopped
- 2 teaspoons fresh dill, chopped
- 4 lettuce leaves
- ½ cup red onion, sliced
- 1 cup tomatoes, chopped

Directions:

1. In a bowl, mix the lemon juice, lemon zest, half of oil, half of garlic, and red pepper.
2. Coat the chicken with the marinade.
3. Marinate it for 1 hour.
4. Toss grated cucumber in salt.

5. Squeeze to release liquid.

6. Add the yogurt, dill, salt, pepper, remaining garlic and remaining oil.

7. Grill the chicken for 4 minutes per side.

8. Shred the chicken and put on top of the lettuce leaves.

9. Top with the yogurt mixture, onion and tomatoes.

10. Wrap the lettuce leaves and secure with a toothpick.

Nutrition Info: Calories 353 Total Fat 9 g Saturated Fat 1 g Cholesterol 58 mg Sodium 559 mg Total Carbohydrate 33 g Dietary Fiber 6 g Total Sugars 6 g Protein 37 g Potassium 459 mg

Spicy Honey Orange Chicken

Servings: 4

Cooking Time: 10 Minutes

Ingredients:

- 1 ½ pounds chicken breast, washed and sliced
- Parsley to taste
- 1 cup coconut, shredded
- ¾ cup breadcrumbs
- 2 whole eggs, beaten
- ½ cup flour
- ½ tsp pepper
- Salt to taste
- ½ cup orange marmalade
- 1 tbsp red pepper flakes
- ¼ cup honey
- 3 tbsp dijon mustard

Directions:

1. Preheat your Air Fryer to 400 F. In a mixing bowl, combine coconut, flour, salt, parsley and pepper. In another bowl, add the beaten eggs. Place breadcrumbs in a third bowl. Dredge chicken in egg mix, flour and finally in the breadcrumbs. Place the chicken in the Air Fryer cooking basket and bake for 15 minutes.

2. In a separate bowl, mix honey, orange marmalade, mustard and pepper flakes. Cover chicken with marmalade mixture and fry for 5 more minutes. Enjoy!

Nutrition Info: Calories: 246; Carbs: 21g; Fat: 6g; Protein: 25g

Crunchy Chicken Fingers

Servings: 2

Cooking Time: 4 Minutes

Ingredients:

- 2 medium-sized chicken breasts, cut in stripes
- 3 tbsp parmesan cheese
- ¼ tbsp fresh chives, chopped
- ⅓ cup breadcrumbs
- 1 egg white
- 2 tbsp plum sauce, optional
- ½ tbsp fresh thyme, chopped
- ½ tbsp black pepper
- 1 tbsp water

Directions:

1. Preheat the Air Fryer to 360 F. Mix the chives, parmesan, thyme, pepper and breadcrumbs. In another bowl, whisk the egg white and mix with the water. Dip the chicken strips into the egg mixture and the breadcrumb mixture. Place the strips in the air fryer basket and cook for 10 minutes. Serve with plum sauce.

Nutrition Info: Calories: 253; Carbs: 31g; Fat: 18g; Protein: 28g

Polynesian Chicken

Servings: 6 Cups

Cooking Time: 4 Hours

Ingredients:

- 3 garlic cloves, minced
- 2 bell peppers, cut into 1/2-inch strips
- 1 (20-ounce) can pineapple chunks in juice, drained, with juice reserved
- 1 1/2-pound boneless chicken breasts, cut into 2-inch cubes
- 1/3 cup honey
- 2 tablespoons tapioca flour
- 3 tablespoons low-sodium soy sauce
- 1 teaspoon ground ginger

Directions:

1. Add reserved pineapple juice, 3 tablespoons of soy sauce, 1/3 cup honey, 1 teaspoon ground ginger and 3 minced cloves of garlic into a bowl; whisk well. Then add 2 tablespoons tapioca flour and whisk again until combined.
2. Add chicken along with chunks of pineapple into a slow cooker.
3. Pour mixture of pineapple juice over chicken and cover the cooker.

4.   Cook for about 4-5 hours on low, until chicken is completely cooked through.

5.   Then add strips of bell pepper in the last hour of cooking. Serve and enjoy!

Nutrition Info: 273 calories; 26 g fat; 37 g total carbs; 26 g protein

Buffalo Chicken

Servings: 8

Cooking Time: 30 Minutes

Ingredients:

- 2 celery stalks, diced
- 1 medium-sized onion, chopped
- 100 ml buffalo wing sauce
- 100 ml chicken broth
- 21 kg chicken breasts, frozen

Directions:

1. Add the celery, onions, wing sauce, chicken broth and chicken to the Instant Pot. Cook frozen chicken on high pressure for 20 minutes. Turn the pressure valve to "Vent" to release all of the pressure.
2. Remove the chicken breasts from the pot, and shred.
3. You can remove most of the liquid from the pot, or not.

Nutrition Info: Calories: 197 Fat: 8g Carbohydrates: 16g Protein: 14g

Chicken & Peanut Stir-fry

Servings: 4

Cooking Time: 15 Minutes

Ingredients:

- 3 tablespoons lime juice
- ½ teaspoon lime zest
- 4 cloves garlic, minced
- 2 teaspoons chili bean sauce
- 1 tablespoon fish sauce
- 1 tablespoon water
- 2 tablespoons peanut butter
- 3 teaspoons oil, divided
- 1 lb. chicken breast, sliced into strips
- 1 red sweet pepper, sliced into strips
- 3 green onions, sliced thinly
- 2 cups broccoli, shredded
- 2 tablespoons peanuts, chopped

Directions:

1. In a bowl, mix the lime juice, lime zest, garlic, chili bean sauce, fish sauce, water and peanut butter.
2. Mix well.
3. In a pan over medium high heat, add 2 teaspoons of oil.

4.   Cook the chicken until golden on both sides.

5.   Pour in the remaining oil.

6.   Add the pepper and green onions.

7.   Add the chicken, broccoli and sauce.

8.   Cook for 2 minutes.

9.   Top with peanuts before serving.

Nutrition Info: Calories 368 Total Fat 11 g Saturated Fat 2 g Cholesterol 66 mg Sodium 556 mg Total Carbohydrate 34 g Dietary Fiber 3 g Total Sugars 4 g Protein 32 g Potassium 482 mg

Meatballs Curry

Servings: 6

Cooking Time: 25 Minutes

Ingredients:

- For Meatballs:
- 1 pound lean ground chicken
- 1 tablespoon onion paste
- 1 teaspoons fresh ginger paste
- 1 teaspoons garlic paste
- 1 green chili, chopped finely
- 1 tablespoon fresh cilantro leaves, chopped
- 1 teaspoon ground coriander
- ½ teaspoon cumin seeds
- ½ teaspoon red chili powder
- ½ teaspoon ground turmeric
- 1/8 teaspoon salt
- For Curry:
- 3 tablespoons olive oil
- ½ teaspoon cumin seeds
- 1 (1-inch) cinnamon stick
- 2 onions, chopped
- 1 teaspoons fresh ginger, minced
- 1 teaspoons garlic, minced
- 4 tomatoes, chopped finely

- 2 teaspoons ground coriander
- 1 teaspoon garam masala powder
- ½ teaspoon ground nutmeg
- ½ teaspoon red chili powder
- ½ teaspoon ground turmeric
- Salt, as required
- 1 cup filtered water
- 3 tablespoons fresh cilantro, chopped

Directions:

1. For meatballs: in a large bowl, add all ingredients and mix until well combined.
2. Make small equal-sized meatballs from mixture.
3. In a large deep skillet, heat the oil over medium heat and cook the meatballs for about 3-5 minutes or until browned from all sides.
4. Transfer the meatballs into a bowl.
5. In the same skillet, add the cumin seeds and cinnamon stick and sauté for about 1 minute.
6. Add the onions and sauté for about 4-5 minutes.
7. Add the ginger and garlic paste and sauté for about 1 minute.
8. Add the tomato and spices and cook, crushing with the back of spoon for about 2-3 minutes.
9. Add the water and meatballs and bring to a boil.
10. Now, reduce the heat to low and simmer for about 10 minutes.

11. Serve hot with the garnishing of cilantro.

12. Meal Prep Tip: Transfer the curry into a large bowl and set aside to cool. Divide the curry into 5 containers evenly. Cover the containers and refrigerate for 1-2 days. Reheat in the microwave before serving.

Nutrition Info: Calories 196 Total Fat 11.4 g Saturated Fat 2.4 g Cholesterol 53 mg Total Carbs 7.9 g Sugar 3.9 g Fiber 2.1 g Sodium 143 mg Potassium 279 mg Protein 16.7 g

Jerk Style Chicken Wings

Servings: 2-3

Cooking Time: 25 Minutes.

Ingredients:

- 1g ground thyme
- 1g dried rosemary
- 2g allspice
- 4g ground ginger
- 3 g garlic powder
- 2g onion powder
- 1g of cinnamon
- 2g of paprika
- 2g chili powder
- 1g nutmeg
- Salt to taste
- 30 ml of vegetable oil
- 0.5 - 1 kg of chicken wings
- 1 lime, juice

Directions:

1. Select Preheat, set the temperature to 200°C and press Start/Pause.
2. Combine all spices and oil in a bowl to create a marinade.

3.   Mix the chicken wings in the marinade until they
     are well covered.

4.   Place the chicken wings in the preheated air
     fryer.

5.   Select Chicken and press Start/Pause. Be sure to
     shake the baskets in the middle of cooking.

6.   Remove the wings and place them on a serving
     plate.

7.   Squeeze fresh lemon juice over the wings and
     serve.

Nutrition Info: Calories: 240 Fat: 15g Carbohydrate: 5g
Protein: 19g Sugars: 4g Cholesterol: 60mg

Italian Chicken

Servings: 4

Cooking Time: 16 Minutes

Ingredients:

- 5 chicken thighs
- 1 tbsp. olive oil
- 1/4 cup parmesan; grated
- 1/2 cup sun dried tomatoes
- 2 garlic cloves; minced
- 1 tbsp. thyme; chopped.
- 1/2 cup heavy cream
- 3/4 cup chicken stock
- 1 tsp. red pepper flakes; crushed
- 2 tbsp. basil; chopped
- Salt and black pepper to the taste

Directions:

1. Season chicken with salt and pepper, rub with half of the oil, place in your preheated air fryer at 350 ºF and cook for 4 minutes.
2. Meanwhile; heat up a pan with the rest of the oil over medium high heat, add thyme garlic, pepper flakes, sun dried tomatoes, heavy cream, stock, parmesan, salt and pepper; stir, bring to a

simmer, take off heat and transfer to a dish that fits your air fryer.

3. Add chicken thighs on top, introduce in your air fryer and cook at 320 °F, for 12 minutes. Divide among plates and serve with basil sprinkled on top.

Nutrition Info: Calories: 272; Fat: 9; Fiber: 12; Carbs: 37; Protein: 23

Coconut Chicken

Servings: 6

Cooking Time: 4 Hours

Ingredients:

- 2 garlic cloves, minced
- Fresh cilantro, minced
- 1/2 cup light coconut milk
- 6 tablespoons sweetened coconut, shredded and toasted
- 2 tablespoons brown sugar
- 6 (about 1-1/2 pounds) boneless skinless chicken thighs
- 2 tablespoons reduced-sodium soy sauce
- 1/8 teaspoon ground cloves

Directions:

1. Mix brown sugar, 1/2 cup light coconut milk, 2 tablespoons soy sauce, 1/8 teaspoon ground cloves and 2 minced cloves of garlic in a bowl.
2. Add 6 chicken boneless thighs into a Crockpot.
3. Now pour the mixture of coconut milk over chicken thighs. Cover the cooker and cook for about 4-5 hours on low.
4. Serve coconut chicken with cilantro and coconut; enjoy!

Nutrition Info: 201 calories; 10 g fat; 6 g total carbs; 21 g protein

Spicy Lime Chicken

Servings: 6

Cooking Time: 3 Hours

Ingredients:

- 3 tablespoons lime juice
- Fresh cilantro leaves
- 1-1/2 pounds (about 4) boneless skinless chicken breast halves
- 1 teaspoon lime zest, grated
- 2 cups chicken broth
- 1 tablespoon chili powder

Directions:

1. Add chicken breast halves into a slow cooker.
2. Add 1 tablespoon chili powder, 3 tablespoons lime juice and 2 cups chicken broth in a small bowl; mix well and pour over chicken.
3. Cover the cooker and cook for about 3 hours on low. Once done, take chicken out from the cooker and let it cool.
4. Once cooled, shred chicken by using forks and transfer back to the Crockpot.
5. Stir in 1 teaspoon grated lime zest. Serve spicy lime chicken with cilantro and enjoy!

Nutrition Info: 132 calories; 3 g fat; 2 g total carbs; 23 g protein

Crock-pot Slow Cooker Ranch Chicken

Servings: 4

Cooking Time: 4 Hours

Ingredients:

- 1 cup chive and onion cream cheese spread
- ½ teaspoon freshly ground black pepper
- 4 boneless chicken breasts
- 1 1-oz package ranch dressing and seasoning mix
- ½ cup low sodium chicken stock

Directions:

1. Spray the Crock-Pot slow cooker with cooking spray and preheat it.
2. Dry chicken with paper towel and transfer it to the Crock-Pot slow cooker.
3. Cook each side, until chicken is browned, for about 4-5 minutes.
4. Add ½ cup low sodium chicken stock, 1 1-oz. package ranch dressing and seasoning mix, 1 cup chive and onion cream cheese spread and ½ teaspoon freshly ground black pepper. Cover the Crock-Pot slow cooker and cook for about 4 hours on Low or until the internal temperature reaches

165 F. Once cooked, take it out from the Crock-Pot slow cooker.

5.   Whisk the sauce present in the Crock-Pot slow cooker until smooth. If you need thick sauce, then cook for about 5-10 minutes, with frequent stirring.

6.   Garnish chicken with sliced onions and bacon and serve.

Nutrition Info: 362 calories; 18.5 g fat; 9.7 g total carbs; 37.3 g protein

Mustard Chicken With Basil

Servings: 4

Cooking Time: 30 Minutes

Ingredients:

- 1 tsp Chicken stock
- 2 Chicken breasts; skinless and boneless chicken breasts: halved
- 1 tbsp Chopped basil
- What you'll need from the store cupboard:
- Salt and black pepper
- 1 tbsp Olive oil
- ½ tsp Garlic powder
- ½ tsp Onion powder
- 1 tsp Dijon mustard

Directions:

1. Press 'Sauté' on the instant pot and add the oil. When it is hot, brown the chicken in it for 2-3 minutes.
2. Mix in the remaining ingredients and seal the lid to cook for 12 minutes at high pressure.
3. Natural release the pressure for 10 minutes, share into plates and serve.

Nutrition Info: Calories 34, fat 3.6, carbs 0.7, protein 0.3, fiber 0.1

Horseradish Meatloaf

Servings: 8

Cooking Time: 45 Minutes

Ingredients:

- 1 ½ lbs. lean ground beef
- 1 egg, beaten
- ½ cup celery, diced fine
- ¼ cup onion, diced fine
- ¼ cup skim milk
- What you'll need from store cupboard:
- 4 slices whole wheat bread, crumbled
- ½ cup ketchup, (chapter 15)
- ¼ cup horseradish
- 2 tbsp. Dijon mustard
- 2 tbsp. chili sauce
- 1 ½ tsp Worcestershire sauce
- ½ tsp salt
- ¼ tsp pepper
- Nonstick cooking spray

Directions:

1. Heat oven to 350 degrees. Spray an 11x7-inch baking dish with cooking spray.
2. In a large bowl, soak bread in milk for 5 minutes. Drain.

3.   Stir in celery, onion, horseradish, mustard, chili
     sauce, Worcestershire, egg, salt, and pepper.
     Crumble beef over mixture and mix well.

4.   Shape into loaf in the prepared baking dish.
     Spread ketchup over the top. Bake 45-50 minutes
     or a meat thermometer reaches 160 degrees. Let
     rest 10 minutes before slicing and serving.

Nutrition Info: Calories 213 Total Carbs 8g Net Carbs 7g
Protein 29g Fat 7g Sugar 2g Fiber 1g

Beef Tenderloin With Roasted Vegetables

Servings: 10

Cooking Time: 1 Hour

Ingredients:

- 3 lb. beef tenderloin
- 1 lb. Yukon gold potatoes, cut in 1-inch wedges
- 1 lb. Brussel sprouts, halved
- 1 lb. baby carrots
- 4 tsp fresh rosemary, diced
- What you'll need from store cupboard:
- ¾ cup dry white wine
- ¾ cup low sodium soy sauce
- 3 cloves garlic, sliced
- 4 tsp Dijon mustard
- 1 ½ tsp ground mustard
- Nonstick cooking spray

Directions:

1. Place beef in a large Ziploc bag.
2. In a small bowl combine wine, soy sauce, rosemary, Dijon, ground mustard, and garlic. Pour half the mixture over the beef. Seal the bag and turn to coat. Refrigerate 4 ½ hours, turning

occasionally. Cover and refrigerate remaining marinade.

3.   Heat oven to 425 degrees. Spray a 9x13-inch baking dish with cooking spray.

4.   Place the potatoes, Brussel sprouts and carrots in the prepared dish. Add reserved marinade and toss to coat. Cover and bake 30 minutes.

5.   Remove tenderloin and discard marinade. Place over vegetables and bake 30-45 minutes or until meat reaches desired doneness.

6.   Remove been and let stand 15 minutes. Check vegetables, if they are not tender bake another 10-15 minutes until done. Slice36 the beef and serve with vegetables.

Nutrition Info: Calories 356 Total Carbs 13g Net Carbs 10g Protein 43g Fat 13g Sugar 4g Fiber 3g

Grilled Tuna Steaks

Servings: 6

Cooking Time: 10 Minutes,

Ingredients:

- 6 6 oz. tuna steaks
- 3 tbsp. fresh basil, diced
- What you'll need from store cupboard:
- 4 ½ tsp olive oil
- ¾ tsp salt
- ¼ tsp pepper
- Nonstick cooking spray

Directions:

1. Heat grill to medium heat. Spray rack with cooking spray.
2. Drizzle both sides of the tuna with oil. Sprinkle with basil, salt and pepper.
3. Place on grill and cook 5 minutes per side, tuna should be slightly pink in the center. Serve.

Nutrition Info: Calories 343 Total Carbs 0g Protein 51g Fat 14g Sugar 0g Fiber 0g

Delicious Fish Tacos

Servings: 8

Cooking Time: 8 Minutes

Ingredients:

- 4 tilapia fillets
- 1/4 cup fresh cilantro, chopped
- 1/4 cup fresh lime juice
- 2 tbsp paprika
- 1 tbsp olive oil
- Pepper
- Salt

Directions:

1. Pour 2 cups of water into the instant pot then place steamer rack in the pot.
2. Place fish fillets on parchment paper.
3. Season fish fillets with paprika, pepper, and salt and drizzle with oil and lime juice.
4. Fold parchment paper around the fish fillets and place them on a steamer rack in the pot.
5. Seal pot with lid and cook on high for 8 minutes.
6. Once done, release pressure using quick release. Remove lid.
7. Remove fish packet from pot and open it.
8. Shred the fish with a fork and serve.

Nutrition Info: Calories 67 Fat 2.5 g Carbohydrates 1.1 g
Sugar 0.2 g Protein 10.8 g Cholesterol 28 mg

Shrimp Coconut Curry

Servings: 2

Cooking Time: 20 Minutes

Ingredients:

- 0.5lb cooked shrimp
- 1 thinly sliced onion
- 1 cup coconut yogurt
- 3tbsp curry paste
- 1tbsp oil or ghee

Directions:

1. Set the Instant Pot to sauté and add the onion, oil, and curry paste.
2. When the onion is soft, add the remaining ingredients and seal.
3. Cook on Stew for 20 minutes.
4. Release the pressure naturally.

Nutrition Info: Calories: 380 Carbs 13; Sugar 4; Fat 22; Protein 40; GL 14

Salmon & Shrimp Stew

Servings: 6

Cooking Time: 21 Minutes

Ingredients:

- 2 tablespoons olive oil
- ½ cup onion, chopped finely
- 2 garlic cloves, minced
- 1 Serrano pepper, chopped
- 1 teaspoon smoked paprika
- 4 cups fresh tomatoes, chopped
- 4 cups low-sodium chicken broth
- 1 pound salmon fillets, cubed
- 1 pound shrimp, peeled and deveined
- 2 tablespoons fresh lime juice
- ¼ cup fresh basil, chopped
- ¼ cup fresh parsley, chopped
- Ground black pepper, as required
- 2 scallions, chopped

Directions:

1. In a large soup pan, melt coconut oil over medium-high heat and sauté the onion for about 5-6 minutes.
2. Add the garlic, Serrano pepper and smoked paprika and sauté for about 1 minute.

3. Add the tomatoes and broth and bring to a gentle simmer over medium heat.
4. Simmer for about 5 minutes.
5. Add the salmon and simmer for about 3-4 minutes.
6. Stir in the remaining seafood and cook for about 4-5 minutes.
7. Stir in the lemon juice, basil, parsley, sea salt and black pepper and remove from heat.
8. Serve hot with the garnishing of scallion.
9. Meal Prep Tip: Transfer the stew into a large bowl and set aside to cool. Divide the stew into 4 containers evenly. Cover the containers and refrigerate for 1-2 days. Reheat in the microwave before serving.

Nutrition Info: Calories 271 Total Fat 11 g Saturated Fat 1.8 g Cholesterol 193 mg Total Carbs 8.6 g Sugar 3.8 g Fiber 2.1 g Sodium 273 mg Potassium 763 mg Protein 34.7 g

Swordfish With Tomato Salsa

Servings: 4

Cooking Time: 12 Minutes

Ingredients:

- 1 cup tomato, chopped
- ¼ cup tomatillo, chopped
- 2 tablespoons fresh cilantro, chopped
- ¼ cup avocado, chopped
- 1 clove garlic, minced
- 1 jalapeño pepper, chopped
- 1 tablespoon lime juice
- Salt and pepper to taste
- 4 swordfish steaks
- 1 clove garlic, sliced in half
- 2 tablespoons lemon juice
- ½ teaspoon ground cumin

Directions:

1. Preheat your grill.
2. In a bowl, mix the tomato, tomatillo, cilantro, avocado, garlic, jalapeño, lime juice, salt and pepper.
3. Cover the bowl with foil and put in the refrigerator.
4. Rub each swordfish steak with sliced garlic.

5.   Drizzle lemon juice on both sides.

6.   Season with salt, pepper and cumin.

7.   Grill for 12 minutes or until the fish is fully
     cooked.

8.   Serve with salsa.

Nutrition Info: Calories 125 g Fat 27.2 g Carbohydrates
13.6 g Protein 7 g Cholesterol 31 mg

Shrimp Boil

Servings: 4

Cooking Time: 15 Minutes

Ingredients:

- 8 oz. raw shrimp, unpeeled
- 8 0oz. chicken sausage, small 1 inch pieces
- 8 oz. baby potatoes
- 1 sliced leek
- 2 corns, cut into half
- What you will need from the store cupboard:
- 3 tablespoons lemon juice
- 10 cups of water
- ¼ cup Old Bay seasoning
- Melted butter
- Lemon wedges

Directions:

1. Bring together the lemon juice, Old Bay, and water in your pot. Boil.
2. Include potatoes and cook for 5-7 minutes.
3. Add the sausage, shrimp, leek, and corn. Cook while stirring for another 5 minutes. The vegetables should be tender and the shrimp must be pink.

4.	Now divide the vegetables, sausage, and shrimp with spoon and tongs among the serving bowls.

5.	Drizzle the cooking liquid equally.

6.	Serve with butter (optional).

Nutrition Info: Calories 202, Carbohydrates 22g, Fiber 2g, Sugar 0g, Cholesterol 109mg, Total Fat 5g, Protein 19g

Shrimp & Artichoke Skillet

Servings: 4

Cooking Time: 10 Minutes

Ingredients:

- 1 ½ cups shrimp, peel & devein
- 2 shallots, diced
- 1 tbsp. margarine
- What you'll need from store cupboard
- 2 12 oz. jars artichoke hearts, drain & rinse
- 2 cups white wine
- 2 cloves garlic, diced fine

Directions:

1. Melt margarine in a large skillet over med-high heat. Add shallot and garlic and cook until they start to brown, stirring frequently.
2. Add artichokes and cook 5 minutes. Reduce heat and add wine. Cook 3 minutes, stirring occasionally.
3. Add the shrimp and cook just until they turn pink. Serve.

Nutrition Info: Calories 487 Total Carbs 26g Net Carbs 17g Protein 64g Fat 5g Sugar 3g Fiber 9g

Red Clam Sauce & Pasta

Servings: 4

Cooking Time: 3 Hours,

Ingredients:

- 1 onion, diced
- ¼ cup fresh parsley, diced
- What you'll need from store cupboard:
- 2 6 ½ oz. cans clams, chopped, undrained
- 14 ½ oz. tomatoes, diced, undrained
- 6 oz. tomato paste
- 2 cloves garlic, diced
- 1 bay leaf
- 1 tbsp. sunflower oil
- 1 tsp Splenda
- 1 tsp basil
- ½ tsp thyme
- ½ Homemade Pasta, cook & drain (chapter 15)

Directions:

1. Heat oil in a small skillet over med-high heat. Add onion and cook until tender, Add garlic and cook 1 minute more. Transfer to crock pot.
2. Add remaining Ingredients, except pasta, cover and cook on low 3-4 hours.
3. Discard bay leaf and serve over cooked pasta.

Nutrition Info: Calories 223 Total Carbs 32g Net Carbs 27g
Protein 12g Fat 6g Sugar 15g Fiber 5g

Grilled Herbed Salmon With Raspberry Sauce & Cucumber Dill Dip

Servings: 4

Cooking Time: 30 Minutes

Ingredients:

- 3 salmon fillets
- 1 tablespoon olive oil
- Salt and pepper to taste
- 1 teaspoon fresh sage, chopped
- 1 tablespoon fresh parsley, chopped
- 2 tablespoons apple juice
- 1 cup raspberries
- 1 teaspoon Worcestershire sauce
- 1 cup cucumber, chopped
- 2 tablespoons light mayonnaise
- ½ teaspoon dried dill

Directions:

1. Coat the salmon fillets with oil.
2. Season with salt, pepper, sage and parsley.
3. Cover the salmon with foil.
4. Grill for 20 minutes or until fish is flaky.

5.   While waiting, mix the apple juice, raspberries and Worcestershire sauce.

6.   Pour the mixture into a saucepan over medium heat.

7.   Bring to a boil and then simmer for 8 minutes.

8.   In another bowl, mix the rest of the ingredients.

9.   Serve salmon with raspberry sauce and cucumber dip.

Nutrition Info: Calories 256 Total Fat 15 g Saturated Fat 3 g Cholesterol 68 mg Sodium 176 mg Total Carbohydrate 6 g Dietary Fiber 1 g Total Sugars 5 g Protein 23 g Potassium 359 mg

Shrimp With Green Beans

Servings: 4

Cooking Time: 2 Minutes

Ingredients:

- ¾ pound fresh green beans, trimmed
- 1 pound medium frozen shrimp, peeled and deveined
- 2 tablespoons fresh lemon juice
- 2 tablespoons olive oil
- Salt and ground black pepper, as required

Directions:

1. Arrange a steamer trivet in the Instant Pot and pour cup of water.
2. Arrange the green beans on top of trivet in a single layer and top with shrimp.
3. Drizzle with oil and lemon juice.
4. Sprinkle with salt and black pepper.
5. Close the lid and place the pressure valve to "Seal" position.
6. Press "Steam" and just use the default time of 2 minutes.
7. Press "Cancel" and allow a "Natural" release.
8. Open the lid and serve.

Nutrition Info: Calories: 223, Fats: 1g, Carbs: 7.9g, Sugar: 1.4g, Proteins: 27.4g, Sodium: 322mg

Cucumber Salad With Pesto

Servings: 4

Cooking Time: 0 Minute

Ingredients:

- 1 cup fresh basil leaves, chopped
- 2 cloves garlic
- 2 tablespoons walnuts
- 1 teaspoon Parmesan cheese
- 1 tablespoon olive oil
- 2 cucumbers, sliced into rounds
- Salt and pepper to taste

Directions:

1. Put the basil, garlic, walnuts, Parmesan cheese and olive oil in a food processor.
2. Pulse until smooth.
3. Season the cucumbers with salt and pepper.
4. Spread pesto on top of each cucumber round.

Nutrition Info: Calories 80 Total Fat 6g Saturated Fat 0.7g Cholesterol 0mg Sodium 4mg Total Carbohydrate 6.5g Dietary Fiber 1.2g Total Sugars 2.6g Protein 2.2g Potassium 266mg

Easy Brussels Sprouts Hash

Servings: 4

Cooking Time: 10 Minutes

Ingredients:

- 3 tablespoons extra-virgin olive oil
- 1 onion, finely chopped
- 1 pound Brussels sprouts, bottoms trimmed off, shredded (see tip)
- ½ teaspoon caraway seeds
- ½ teaspoon sea salt
- ⅛ teaspoon freshly ground black pepper
- ¼ cup red wine vinegar
- 1 tablespoon Dijon mustard
- 1 tablespoon honey
- 3 garlic cloves, minced

Directions:

1. In a large skillet over medium-high heat, heat the olive oil until it shimmers.
2. Add the onion, Brussels sprouts, caraway seeds, sea salt, and pepper. Cook for 7 to 10 minutes, stirring occasionally, until the Brussels sprouts begin to brown.

3.   While the Brussels sprouts cook, whisk the vinegar, mustard, and honey in a small bowl and set aside.

4.   Add the garlic to the skillet and cook for 30 seconds, stirring constantly.

5.   Add the vinegar mixture to the skillet. Cook for about 5 minutes, stirring, until the liquid reduces by half.

Nutrition Info: Calories: 176; Protein: 11g; Total Carbohydrates: 19g; Sugars: 8g; Fiber: 5g; Total Fat: 11g; Saturated Fat: 1g; Cholesterol: 0mg; Sodium: 309mg

Vegetable And Bean Stew

Servings: 6

Cooking Time: 20 Minutes

Ingredients:

- 1 lb. potatoes, cut into small 1 inch chunks
- 2 parsnips, 1-inch chunks
- 2 carrots, 1-inch chunks
- 19 oz. pinto beans, drained and rinsed
- 1 acorn squash
- What you will need from the store cupboard:
- 2 teaspoons olive oil
- 1 cup apple cider
- 1 cup vegetable broth, low-sodium
- Salt and pepper to taste

Directions:

1. Preheat your oven to 350 ºF.
2. Divide the squash. Remove the seeds. Cut the flesh into 4 cm chunks and peel the skin.
3. Put them in a bowl and also the carrots, potatoes, and parsnips.
4. Drizzle olive oil. Toss well to coat.
5. Now stir the garlic in. Season with pepper and salt lightly.
6. Keep the rosemary sprigs in your roasting pan.

7.   Spread vegetables in a single layer on top.

8.   Roast to brown lightly. Turn once.

9.   Take out from the oven. Stir the cider, broth and pinto beans in.

10.   Use foil to cover your pan tightly.

11.   Cook until your vegetables have become tender.

12.   Garnish with rosemary sprigs.

Nutrition Info: Calories 278, Fat 3g, Protein 8g, Carbohydrates 58g, Fiber 11g, Cholesterol 0mg, Sugar 0.6g

Grilled Zucchini With Tomato Relish

Servings: 4

Cooking Time: 10 Minutes

Ingredients:

- 1 lb. zucchini, sliced in half
- 1 tablespoon olive oil
- Salt and pepper to taste
- 1 teaspoon red wine vinegar
- 1 tablespoon mint, chopped
- 1 cup tomatoes, chopped

Directions:

1. Preheat your grill.
2. Brush both sides of zucchini with oil and season with salt and pepper.
3. Grill for 3 to 4 minutes per side.
4. In a bowl, mix the rest of the ingredients with the remaining oil.
5. Season with salt and pepper.
6. Spread tomato relish on top of the grilled zucchini before serving.

Nutrition Info: Calories 71 Total Fat 5 g Saturated Fat 1 g Cholesterol 0 mg Sodium 157 mg Total Carbohydrate 6 g

Dietary Fiber 2 g Total Sugars 4 g Protein 2 g Potassium 413 mg

Carrot Soup With Tempeh

Servings: 6

Cooking Time: 45 Minutes

Ingredients:

- ¼ cup olive oil, divided
- 1 large yellow onion, chopped
- Salt, to taste
- 2 pounds' carrots, peeled, and cut into ½-inch rounds
- 2 tablespoons fresh dill, chopped
- 4½ cups homemade vegetable broth
- 12 ounces' tempeh, cut into ½-inch cubes
- ¼ cup tomato paste
- 1 teaspoon fresh lemon juice

Directions:

1. In a large soup pan, heat 2 tablespoons of the oil over medium heat and cook the onion with salt for about 6–8 minutes, stirring frequently.
2. Add the carrots and stir to combine.
3. Lower the heat to low and cook, covered for about 5 minutes, stirring frequently.
4. Add in the broth and bring to a boil over high heat.

5.   Lower the heat to a low and simmer, covered for
     about 30 minutes.
6.   Meanwhile, in a skillet, heat the remaining oil
     over medium-high heat and cook the tempeh for
     about 3–5 minutes.
7.   Stir in the dill and cook for about 1 minute.
8.   Remove from the heat.
9.   Remove the pan of soup from heat and stir in
     tomato paste and lemon juice.
10.   With an immersion blender, blend the soup until
      smooth and creamy.
11.   Serve the soup hot with the topping of tempeh.

Nutrition Info: Calories 294 Total Fat 15.7 g Saturated Fat
2.8 g Cholesterol 0 mg Sodium 723 mg Total Carbs 25.9 g
Fiber 4.9 g Sugar 10.4 g Protein 16.4 g

Beet Soup

Servings: 2

Cooking Time: 5 Minutes

Ingredients:

- 2 cups coconut yogurt
- 4 teaspoons fresh lemon juice
- 2 cups beets, trimmed, peeled, and chopped
- 2 tablespoons fresh dill
- Salt, to taste
- 1 tablespoon pumpkin seeds
- 2 tablespoons coconut cream
- 1 tablespoon fresh chives, minced

Directions:

1. In a high-speed blender, add all ingredients and pulse until smooth.
2. Transfer the soup into a pan over medium heat and cook for about 3–5 minutes or until heated through.
3. Serve immediately with the garnishing of chives and coconut cream.

Nutrition Info: Calories 230 Total Fat 8 g Saturated Fat 5.8 g Cholesterol 0 mg Sodium 218 mg Total Carbs 33.5 g Fiber 4.2 g Sugar 27.5 g Protein 8 g

Balsamic Roasted Carrots

Servings: 4

Cooking Time: 30 Minutes

Ingredients:

- 1½ pounds carrots, quartered lengthwise
- 2 tablespoons extra-virgin olive oil
- ¼ teaspoon sea salt
- ⅛ teaspoon freshly ground black pepper
- 3 tablespoons balsamic vinegar

Directions:

1. Preheat the oven to 425°F.
2. In a large bowl, toss the carrots with the olive oil, sea salt, and pepper. Place in a single layer in a roasting pan or on a rimmed baking sheet. Roast for 20 to 30 minutes until the carrots are caramelized.
3. Toss with the vinegar and serve.

Nutrition Info: Calories: 132; Protein: 1g; Total Carbohydrates: 17g; Sugars: 8g; Fiber: 4g; Total Fat: 7g; Saturated Fat: 1g; Cholesterol: 0mg; Sodium: 235mg

Roasted Lemon Mixed Vegetables

Servings: 5

Cooking Time: 20 Minutes

Ingredients:

- 2 teaspoons lemon zest
- 1-1/2 cups broccoli florets
- 1-1/2 cups cauliflower florets
- 1 teaspoon oregano, crushed
- ¾ cup red bell pepper, diced
- What you will need from the store cupboard:
- 1 tablespoon olive oil
- 2 sliced garlic cloves
- ¼ teaspoon salt

Directions:

1. Preheat your oven to 350 ºF.
2. Bring together the broccoli, garlic, and cauliflower in a baking pan.
3. Drizzle oil. Sprinkle the salt and oregano.
4. Roast for 10 minutes.
5. Now add the bell pepper to the vegetables. Stir and combine.
6. Roast until the vegetables have become light brown and crisp.

7.   Sprinkle lemon zest and serve.

Nutrition Info: Calories 52, Carbohydrates 5g, Fiber 2g, Cholesterol 0mg, Fat 3g, Sugar 0.2g, Protein 2g, Sodium 134mg

Butternut Fritters

Servings: 6

Cooking Time: 15 Minutes

Ingredients:

- 5 cup butternut squash, grated
- 2 large eggs
- 1 tablespoon. fresh sage, diced fine
- 2/3 cup flour
- 2 tablespoons olive oil
- Salt and pepper, to taste

Directions:

1. Heat oil in a large skillet over med-high heat.
2. In a large bowl, combine squash, eggs, sage and salt and pepper to taste. Fold in flour.
3. Drop ¼ cup mixture into skillet, keeping fritters at least 1 inch apart. Cook till golden brown on both sides, about 2 minutes per side.
4. Transfer to paper towel lined plate. Repeat. Serve immediately with your favorite dipping sauce.

Nutrition Info: Calories 164 Total Carbohydrates 24g Net Carbohydrates 21g Protein 4g Fat 6g Sugar 3g Fiber 3g

Mushroom Toast

Servings: 8

Cooking Time: 10 Minutes

Ingredients:

- 1 lb. button mushrooms
- 2 tablespoons thyme, chopped
- 3 tablespoons parsley, chopped
- 2 celery stalks, chopped
- 8 whole-grain bread slices, 1-inch slices
- What you will need from the store cupboard:
- 2 tablespoons sour cream, low-fat
- 1 crushed garlic clove
- ½ cup ricotta cheese
- Pinch of cayenne pepper
- Salt and pepper to taste

Directions:

1. Keep the celery, ricotta, cayenne pepper and parsley in a bowl. Mix well.
2. Preheat your oven to 350 °F.
3. Halve the large mushrooms. Place them in a big skillet.
4. Add the thyme, garlic, sour cream, and 1 teaspoon of water.

5.   Cook covered until your mushrooms have become
      tender.
6.   Season with pepper and salt.
7.   In the meantime, toast both sides of the bread
      slices.
8.   Apply ricotta mixture on one side of the toast.
      Cut it in half.
9.   Place toasts on serving plates.
10.   Now spoon the mushroom mixture over them
      before serving.

Nutrition Info: Calories 148, Carbohydrates 24g, Fiber 4g,
Cholesterol 6mg, Sugar 0.3g, Fat 4g, Protein 8g

Irish Stew

Servings: 2

Cooking Time: 35 Minutes

Ingredients:

- 1.5lb diced lamb shoulder
- 1lb chopped vegetables
- 1 cup low sodium beef broth
- 3 minced onions
- 1tbsp ghee

Directions:

1. Mix all the ingredients in your Instant Pot.
2. Cook on Stew for 35 minutes.
3. Release the pressure naturally.

Nutrition Info: Calories: 330; Carbs: 9; Sugar: 2; Fat: 12; Protein: 49; GL: 3

Vegetarian Split Pea Soup In A Crock Pot

Servings: 8

Cooking Time: 10 Minutes

Ingredients:

- 2 chopped ribs celery
- 2 cubes low-sodium bouillon
- 8 c. water
- 2 c. uncooked green split peas
- 3 bay leaves
- 2 carrots
- 2 chopped potatoes
- Pepper and salt

Directions:

1. In your Crock-Pot, put the bouillon cubes, split peas, and water. Stir a bit to break up the bouillon cubes.
2. Next, add the chopped potatoes, celery, and carrots followed with bay leaves.
3. Stir to combine well.
4. Cover and cook for at least 4 hours on your Crock-Pot's low setting or until the green split peas are soft.

5.   Add a bit salt and pepper as needed.

6.   Before serving, remove the bay leaves and enjoy.

Nutrition Info: Calories: 149, Fat:1 g, Carbs:30 g, Protein:7 g, Sugars:3 g, Sodium:732 mg

Thai Peanut, Carrot, & Shrimp Soup

Servings: 4

Cooking Time: 10 Minutes

Ingredients:

- 3 garlic cloves, minced
- ½ onion, sliced
- 1 tablespoon Thai red curry paste
- 1 tablespoon coconut oil
- fresh cilantro, minced, for garnish
- ½ pound shrimp, peeled and deveined
- ½ cup unsweetened plain almond milk
- 4 cups of low-sodium vegetable broth
- ½ cup whole unsalted peanuts
- 2 cups carrots, chopped

Directions:

1. In a pan, heat your oil over medium-high heat until shimmering.

2. Add your curry paste to the pan and cook continually stirring for about 1 minute. Add the garlic, onion, and carrots, along with peanuts to the pan. Continue cooking for 3 minutes or until your onion begins to soften.

3. Add your broth and bring to a boil. Reduce heat to a low setting and simmer for 6 minutes or until carrots are tender.

4. Use your immersion blender to puree your soup until smooth and return to pot. With heat setting on low, add the almond milk and stir to combine. Add your shrimp to the pot and cook for 3 minutes or until cooked.

5. Garnish soup with cilantro, then serve and enjoy!

Nutrition Info: Carbs per serving: 17g

Ham Asparagus Soup

Servings: 3-4

Cooking Time: 55 Min.

Ingredients:

- 5 crushed garlic cloves
- 1 cup chopped ham
- 4 cups (preferably homemade) chicken broth
- 2 pounds trimmed and halved asparagus spears
- 2 tablespoons butter
- 1 chopped yellow onion
- ½ teaspoon dried thyme
- Salt and freshly (finely ground) black pepper, as per taste preference

Directions:

1. Arrange Instant Pot over a dry platform in your kitchen. Open its top lid and switch it on.
2. Find and press "SAUTE" cooking function; add the butter in it and allow it to heat.
3. In the pot, add the onions; cook (while stirring) until turns translucent and softened for around 4-5 minutes.
4. Add the garlic, ham bone and broth; stir, and cook for about 2-3 minutes.
5. Add the other ingredients; gently stir to mix well.

6.   Close the lid to create a locked chamber; make sure that safety valve is in locking position.

7.   Find and press "SOUP" cooking function; timer to 45 minutes with default "HIGH" pressure mode.

8.   Allow the pressure to build to cook the ingredients.

9.   After cooking time is over press "CANCEL" setting. Find and press "QPR" cooking function. This setting is for quick release of inside pressure.

10.   Slowly open the lid, add the mix in a blender or processor.

11.   Blend or process to make a smooth mix. Place the mix in serving bowls and enjoy the keto.

Nutrition Info: Calories - 146 Fat: 7g Saturated Fat: 3g Trans Fat: 0g Carbohydrates: 5g Fiber: 4g Sodium: 262mg Protein: 10g

Cabbage Soup

Servings: 2

Cooking Time: 35 Minutes

Ingredients:

- 1lb shredded cabbage
- 1 cup low sodium vegetable broth
- 1 shredded onion
- 2tbsp mixed herbs
- 1tbsp black pepper

Directions:

1. Mix all the ingredients in your Instant Pot.
2. Cook on Stew for 35 minutes.
3. Release the pressure naturally.

Nutrition Info: Calories: 60; Carbs: 2; Sugar: 0; Fat: 2; Protein: 4; GL: 1

Chickpea Soup

Servings: 2

Cooking Time: 35 Minutes

Ingredients:

- 1lb cooked chickpeas
- 1lb chopped vegetables
- 1 cup low sodium vegetable broth
- 2tbsp mixed herbs

Directions:

1. Mix all the ingredients in your Instant Pot.
2. Cook on Stew for 35 minutes.
3. Release the pressure naturally.

Nutrition Info: Calories: 310; Carbs: 20; Sugar: 3; Fat: 5; Protein: 27; GL: 5

Meatball Stew

Servings: 2

Cooking Time: 25 Minutes

Ingredients:

- 1lb sausage meat
- 2 cups chopped tomato
- 1 cup chopped vegetables
- 2tbsp Italian seasonings
- 1tbsp vegetable oil

Directions:

1. Roll the sausage into meatballs.
2. Put the Instant Pot on Sauté and fry the meatballs in the oil until brown.
3. Mix all the ingredients in your Instant Pot.
4. Cook on Stew for 25 minutes.
5. Release the pressure naturally.

Nutrition Info: Calories: 300; Carbs: 4; Sugar: 1; Fat: 12; Protein: 40; GL: 2

Squash Soup

Servings: 6

Cooking Time: 8 Hours

Ingredients:

- 2 lb butternut squash, peeled, chopped into chunks
- 1 tsp ginger, minced
- 1/4 tsp cinnamon
- 1 Tbsp curry powder
- 2 bay leaves
- 1 tsp black pepper
- 1/2 cup heavy cream
- 2 cups chicken stock
- 1 Tbsp garlic, minced
- 2 carrots, cut into chunks
- 2 apples, peeled, cored and diced
- 1 large onion, diced
- 1 tsp salt

Directions:

1. Spray a crock pot inside with cooking spray.
2. Add all ingredients except cream to the crock pot and stir well.
3. Cover and cook on low for 8 hours.

4.   Purée the soup using an immersion blender until smooth and creamy.

5.   Stir in heavy cream and season soup with pepper and salt.

6.   Serve and enjoy.

Nutrition Info: Calories 170 Fat 4.4 g Carbohydrates 34.4 g Sugar 13.4g Protein 2.9 g Cholesterol 14 mg

Spinach & Basil Chicken Soup

Servings: 4

Cooking Time: 10 Minutes

Ingredients:

- 1 cup spinach
- 2 cups cooked and shredded chicken
- 4 cups chicken broth
- 1 cup cheddar cheese, shredded
- 4 ounces' cream cheese
- ½ tsp chili powder
- ½ tsp ground cumin
- ½ tsp fresh parsley, chopped
- Salt and black pepper, to taste

Directions:

1. In a pot, add the chicken broth and spinach, bring to a boil and cook for 5-8 minutes. Transfer to a food processor, add in the cream cheese and pulse until smooth. Return the mixture to a pot and place over medium heat. Cook until hot, but do not bring to a boil.
2. Add chicken, chili powder, and cumin and cook for about 3-5 minutes, or until it is heated through.

3. Stir in cheddar cheese and season with salt and
    pepper. Serve hot in bowls sprinkled with parsley.

Nutrition Info: Calories 351, Fat: 22.4g, Net Carbs: 4.3g,
Protein: 21.6g

www.ingramcontent.com/pod-product-compliance
Lightning Source LLC
Chambersburg PA
CBHW070744030726
47601CB00001B/143